Feelings

And

Thoughts

Of

The

Enemy

Depression is of the devil, the enemy!

It's just like stress, it's a silent killer!

The enemy use's this decease to squeeze your mind dry!

The enemy wants to empty everything good in your mind out!

He wants to squeeze your mind like a tube of tooth paste.

He sends his thoughts in hopes of killing you, destroying you and stealing your mind.

He will send images to you that are not real. He will mess with your nerves and make you feel like you're crazy at times

Your mind is his battle ground.

He will use this decease to make you feel like no one cares for you.

No one wants to help you.

He will make you feel isolated from everyone.

He will have you feeling like everything kind of noise there is irritates you.

Every interest that you have ever had he will take it away from you.

He will pull your mind apart from reality

If the enemy can take compete control of your mind, he will have you.

The enemy will have your mind unstable.

He'll have you all out of wrack.

Depression will have you feeling sick all the time in your mind.

This is a feeling from the enemy.

The enemy will use this decease to make you feel like giving up on everything you believe in.

He will use depression to make you feel lazy at times.

You don't want to go anywhere, or talk to anyone.

Depression will block your focus from where you're going.

The devil tried to destroy me, but he didn't succeed and he never will.

These feeling and thoughts I'm talking about, I went through them.

Yes! He was squeezing me like a tube of tooth paste!

I am connected to the vine!

I have a personal relationship with Jesus Christ.

I am redeemed by the blood of the Lamb!

No weapon formed against me shall prosper!

I know that it will come, but it will not destroy me, why because Jesus Christ is my defender.

When the enemy sends these thoughts and feelings of his in your mind, where's what you do! Put the word on him! Put Prayer on him! Put your feet on the devil's neck! Make him take his filthy hands off you!

The enemy's plan is to expose you for not being who you say that you are in Christ Jesus! Be like Job and hold on, no matter what may come or go you hold on to Jesus!!!

Lucifer wants to expose you, but you need to expose him!

He is the father of darkness and that's why he use's depression in a person's life to make everything look dark! He wants to take your hope!

Light is more powerful then darkness! Stay in the light it will save your life! Keep walking upright before God!

Keep letting your light shine!!

Listen if Jesus healed all those decease's when he walked the earth over some 2000 years ago; He can still heal those same deceases today!! Depression didn't just appear today it's been around for some time, and it's nothing new to God!

Don't let this darkness take over your mind!

Go see your doctor to get treated. That's why God put doctor here to help out in cases like this. God was thinking about all those deceases and knew that they would be around until the end. He said let me put doctors on the earth so that I can work though them also to heal my people.

If you feel like you need to take a break from everything and get some rest let your doctor know. Let your family members know what you're dealing so that they can be a support for you!

When I first found out years ago that I was suffering from depression, I really didn't understand what it was. All I knew was I wanted to feel better. I had to send my baby to stay with the sitter a few nights and I didn't like that.

I learned how to stay busy to keep my mind occupied, but that caught up with me. It will burn you out if you're not careful.

My doctor sat me up for some group therapy sessions and they really helped me. I forgot that didn't have to go through this alone and you don't neither.

Turn your feelings into joyous feelings!

Turn your thoughts into powerful thoughts!

JESUS IS THE ANSWER TO ALL OUR NEEDS!!!

Read healing scriptures each day!

Take time to listen to preaching tapes if you're not a member of a church! Go to YouTube and pull up some preaching videos!

You can't get through this alone you will need a higher power and you don't have it apart from Jesus!

Depression is a sickness that will cause you to hurt yourself or do bodily harm to yourself.

Get the help you need today?

Jesus has done it for me and he can do it for you if you let him in your heart today!

You have a bright future don't let the enemy steal it away from you!

You have a story to tell and the devil wants to keep you quite in that dark room of your mind!

Take a bold stand against the enemy and let the light in your mind!

The enemy will make you feel like nothing is working out for you.

He will have you acting in a way that you don't normally act.

Depression is a mood disorder!

That's it! Oh man! Depression will have you feeling all kinds of ways.

Many Americans around the world are suffering from this sickness.

See a doctor before it's too late!

Look up the symptoms of depression if you feel like you have it!

If you identify with several of the following signs and symptoms—
especially the first two—and they just won't go away, you may be
suffering from depression.

- you feel hopeless and helpless
- you've lost interest in friends, activities, and things you used
  to enjoy
- you feel tired all the time
- your sleep and appetite has changed
- you can't concentrate or find that previously easy tasks are
  now difficult
- you can't control your negative thoughts, no matter how
  much you try
- you are much more irritable, short-tempered, or aggressive
  than usual

Depression is a major risk factor for suicide. The deep despair and hopelessness that goes along with depression can make suicide feel like the only way to escape the pain. If you have a loved one with depression, take any suicidal talk or behavior seriously and watch for the warning signs:

- Talking about killing or harming one's self
- Expressing strong feelings of hopelessness or being trapped
- An unusual preoccupation with death or dying
- Acting recklessly, as if they have a death wish (e.g. speeding through red lights)
- Calling or visiting people to say goodbye
- Getting affairs in order (giving away prized possessions, tying up loose ends)
- Saying things like "Everyone would be better off without me" or "I want out"
- A sudden switch from being extremely depressed to acting calm and happy

Don't play with this seek help right away! This is what the enemy wants you to do! Then he wins the game!

It's hard for me to concentrate on simple things now, all I do is relax and get focused on what I trying to do. If I get irritated with it, I leave it and come back to it later.

Sleep is something I could not do for a while! I could not work at one time; I just didn't want to do anything. I stopped going to church because the music was bothering me. Lord knows I went through the ringer with this demon!

I have never suffered from anything like this before in my entire life until after I had my baby at age 38.

I remember feeling like cold water was running inside my ankles.

I was feeling like I couldn't breathe, I thought that I was going to drop dead at any moment! It took the doctors in the ER a while to figure out what was going on with me. When I told them that I had just had a baby, they knew then that it was depression!

It took me a while to get back to normal, but it happened!

I didn't make it this far on my own. I have my church family, and I finally told my baby sister and here's what she said to me in a text.

You already know that is a trick from the enemy!

You belong to the most high God! You don't belong to the devil! You have the most high King in you! Now call Jesus!!!

She was reminding me of who I am in Jesus Christ!

I pray that my testimony help set someone free from the grips of this demon call depression.

Other Books by the Author

I give you strength Peace Hope and Joy

YouTube classroom

On

Amazon

www.ingramcontent.com/pod-product-compliance
Lightning Source LLC
Chambersburg PA
CBHW071327310526
45789CB00016B/1680